EVERY DAY MINDFULNESS
IN SCHOOLS

Every Day Mindfulness in Schools

An Educator's Guide

CHRIS MAXWELL

Edinburgh Publishing

Contents

To my teaching friends and colleagues all over the world.
I hope this goes some way to making your lives a little easier.

To all the students I have taught over the years, thank you for being my biggest teachers.

Introduction

It seems like mindfulness is the word on everyone's lips at the moment. Almost every time we turn on the TV or go online someone somewhere is promoting it. From celebrities to sports stars, entrepreneurs to politicians it seems like everyone is doing it.

The benefits of mindfulness have been well documented but it is important to be aware that mindfulness is not a "cure all." There is now, though, some compelling evidence to suggest that it can influence people's health, well-being and happiness when practised regularly - and that includes children. Mindful.org (Reference 1) identify some of the proven benefits which include:

- Better focus and concentration
- Improved sleep
- Decrease in stress, anxiety and depression
- Improved self-control
- Increased compassion
- Reduces disruptive behaviour

So, what is mindfulness? In simple terms mindfulness is being present in the moment. According to Mindful.org.

"Mindfulness is the basic human ability to be fully present, aware of where we are and what we're doing, and not overly reactive or be overwhelmed by what's going on around us."

Possibly the most quoted definition is by Jon Kabat-Zinn a mindfulness guru, author and long-term advocate of mindfulness. He is the person who introduced mindfulness for stress reduction to the western world.

"Mindfulness is awareness that arises through paying attention, on purpose, in the present moment, and non-judgmentally."

Mindfulness is all very well, but is this just something else that teachers need to shoe-horn into an already over-crowded curriculum? The good news is, no! Mindfulness can be incorporated into many of the daily activities that already take place in schools and classrooms across the country and indeed the world.

Mindfulness doesn't have to be a sit down, cross legged, meditation with our eyes closed and finger and thumb touching together.

I guarantee though that there will be at least one child or colleague who strikes that pose when you mention the word mindfulness!

Wouldn't it be better if mindfulness techniques were something that we all have in our toolkits? Something we could go to without fuss, that doesn't take too long, is in-expensive or even free.

I'm not suggesting that mindfulness is a "fix all" but it's definitely something that when practised regularly can make a big difference. Even with children who are reluctant at first, you'll often find that over time, if you keep it low key and don't engage with avoidance or low-level disruption, they begin to take part. If you're interested in learning some skills and techniques...Read on!

I'm often asked about the difference between mindfulness and meditation? They certainly have qualities that overlap but perhaps a simplified way to explain this is that meditation is usually a more formal practice, with an intention. It is most often a seated practice. There are many different forms of meditation including loving kindness, mantra and visualisation meditations. Mindfulness is being present in the here and now and can be both formal and informal. It is paying attention to and noticing what is happening around and within you in the present moment.

Some of the meditations in this book are available on the Insight Timer App. Both the app and meditations are free. (Reference 2)

Chapter 1

The School Day

By the time they get to school many young people, and indeed parents, will have experienced the early morning rush to get out of the house. The repeated shouts of,

"I can't find..." "Have you got...?" "Don't forget..." "Where's my...?" will be echoing through almost every house in the land, and that's before they start on the journey to school. For those who walk, cycle or scoot to school they'll have negotiated commuters in cars and on foot, all desperate to get to where they're going to as quickly as possible, many with little thought or care for the young people around them. And then there's those who are driven to school. The repeated shouts of,

"If you're not in the car in five minutes, I'm going without you!" "Eat your toast on the way we haven't got time to waste."

Familiar to many of us I know.

No wonder then that when they reach school, many young people are not ready to learn. Their heads are full of trying to make sense of how they even got to school and that's before we take into account the traumatic Adverse Childhood Experiences (ACE) that some have had to deal with at home. No wonder that anxiety and school refusal is on the rise. Many young people have experienced stress before they even get through the school gates.

Wouldn't it be great to have something up your sleeve, one or two tried and tested techniques, that you can build into the school day? The good news is - you do! And like everything else the more you do it, the more benefits you'll see as it becomes second nature. Don't take my word for it though. Get started and see for yourself.

Obviously, when you are teaching these skills, you will be aware of the age and stage of the young people you are teaching and the presentation of the skills and vocabulary will be appropriate for their level of understanding. You are the experts in the age group you're teaching and you also know your school and young people better than anyone else. As you begin to use these techniques more and more you will gain confidence in adapting them for yourself and the needs of your class or group. Don't be afraid to combine some of the skills and techniques and do ask the young people which bits they like/dislike, how they feel, where they feel it, and whether it feels different from the first time/last time. Practising mindfulness can be a rewarding experience for both the teacher and students. You and they aren't going to like every mindfulness practice that you do but what a gift to give young people. It's a toolkit that they can come back to, pick and choose what they need for different times and have the confidence and understanding to use the techniques throughout their lives. I promise with a little commitment and very little extra time in the beginning, mindfulness will become as natural to your daily routine as break time.

Chapter 2

Lining Up and Counting

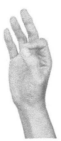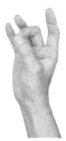

Some schools line young people up in the playground before the school day begins, while others are more informal and the classroom is open to drop bags off or just stay in. Whichever method your school uses, there will be times when you need your class or group to line up, maybe for moving around school safely, out on a trip or going to lunch. As we know this can be a flash point for some, those who find it hard to stand still, can't help poking or annoying the person in front or behind them and end up in all kinds of trouble from both their peers and you. Counting to four mindfully can be an absolute game changer and once they've learned the technique it's a transferable skill that you and they can use in almost any situation. I have used this technique many times with both young people and adults and even the youngest pre-schoolers are desperate to show that they can count to four. The trick is counting slowly and it's best taught when the class are settled, perhaps on the carpet in front of you or at their desks.

How to do it – first ask the children if they have ever been worried, scared, angry, upset or unable to sleep. Usually this results in a show of hands for almost every emotion and it helps if you share that this happens to you and other adults too. Explain that these are normal emotions which we all experience at different times, even adults. Then explain that you are going to teach them how to do something that will help them to feel calmer when this happens. If the children are very young ask them if they can count to four – they love to tell you that,

"Of course, we can, that's easy!"

With very young children you might want to do a little practise, they love to show you that they can! Next ask them to put their hands up in front of themselves, palms facing their face. Then slowly, and with each count, tap your finger tip to the tip of your thumb (starting with index finger, middle finger, ring finger, little finger). The slower the better and do slow them down if they start to speed up. You'll notice after even two or three rounds that everything calms down, it may take longer for some but the more you do it the more it will become a quick go-to strategy that works.

That's all very well with younger children but young people and teens are less likely to want to engage with this without some adaptations. The principles remain the same, slow counting to four but suggest doing the counting and finger taps down by their side so no one can see. Another suggestion is if they are sitting in a lesson and feeling anxious or upset, they can rest their hand on the desk or table and gently tap their fingers one at a time while counting to four in their heads. They can do this, with practice, during an assessment or exam or even with their hands in their pockets, again so that they don't feel self-conscious. It's also a good antidote to those who have a tendency to poke or otherwise provoke those around them! Once you have got their attention and understanding of the concept then link breathing into it. So, breathe in as you count one, breathe out as you count two, breathe in as you count three and breathe out as you count four. I call this Count to Calm on Insight Timer (Reference 3).

-

Chapter 3

Grounding

Young people who aren't grounded can feel out of sorts in so many ways. They won't say of course – "I'm not grounded" - but it will be displayed in their behaviour and body language; the way they can't settle to a task, withdraw from an activity or become completely over the top. Young children especially have an innate need to move and when doing so they use up energy and naturally ground themselves. Many young people today spend less time running and playing outside, their lives can be quite sedentary. Previous generations played outside, running free, taking risks with minimal adult supervision. Now their lives tend to be spent more indoors or in organised activities that involve a lot more adult direction and planning. Subsequently, many young people arrive in school not able to settle to learn. It's always a good idea to have some kind of movement session, however short before you expect them to sit down and listen. Many teachers already do this with movement breaks, encouraging the whole class to stand up and move, dance, shake and jump at regular intervals. There are also some excellent YouTube videos that young people love to join in with. Experiment with all these – it only needs to be for a couple of minutes before, during or after each lesson, but the benefits are enormous. Another useful strategy can be to stand behind their seat resting their hands on the back of the chair. Ask them to feel their feet on the floor, really pushing down, feeling their leg muscles getting stronger. Then ask them to use their hands to push down on the back of the seat. Get them to experiment with different degrees of pressure. How does it make them feel? Where do they feel it; top of their arms, legs or somewhere else? Can they feel their energy? This is a good one to do between transitions, it's quick and easy and they're getting up anyway. It's also good to do at the start of each lesson whether or not they're staying in the same room. If it's practised regularly, it can signal the start of the next lesson, a preparation to learn.

Chapter 4

Mindful Movement
and Walking

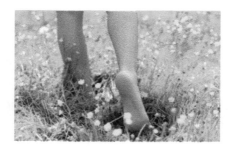

As previously mentioned, movement is vital for young people and movement breaks and grounding are essential for enabling them to focus and learn. This is definitely one area where you need to be aware of age and stage of those you are teaching. Try some of these exercises with a class of teens and you may find yourself wishing you hadn't! Most younger children however respond well and you never know, you may even have a class of teens who actually enjoy this too.

Most of the mindful movement exercises can be done in the classroom. If you're feeling brave and don't mind fastening thirty sets of shoe laces after, then they can do it in socks or bare feet! As with all things mindful it's about being present in exactly what they are doing, really noticing and feeling each movement. It's good to get them grounded from the outset and 'the behind the desk or chair' activity, previously mentioned, is a good way to start. Explain to them that they are going to be moving slowly and very quietly, not exercising just moving. Younger children love the idea of doing something in slow motion. Start by asking them to notice their feet on the ground – depending if they have socks or shoes on ask them to think about whether the floor is warm or cold. Encourage them to spread their toes out wide if they can. Introduce an element of play, there's no reason why this can't be fun. Try something like – "This floor is made of..." Get them to think what it would feel, sound, smell, look like if they were walking in whatever; sand, mud, jelly anything you or they can think of. Let them exaggerate the movement. * Be aware of children who are neurodivergent as they may find this exercise and some of the other exercises quite challenging. Often, they have sensory issues which may trigger a response. As with everything in this book, you know the children in your care best and will be able to adapt or work around the suggestions on offer. Talk about what their toes and feet and ankles feel like and then the different parts of their legs. Like adults, young people don't always notice. They take things for granted but it can be a useful tool later if they can identify what they feel and where. Be conscious of the breath during this exercise and if they have already used the Count to Calm exercise encourage them to use the breathing. Ask them to notice if their breath changes while they are moving, even though the exercise is slow. You can add all kinds of movement, be playful and go with the flow. There isn't any right or wrong way other than to keep it slow and mindful. Sometimes if young people are finding it hard to do this, they may need a more vigorous form of exercise to help them settle. If you're close to the playground a quick run around should work. But if you are in the classroom some running on the spot, jumping or toe touching can be enough to reduce the excess energy before starting the mindful movement.

Move slowly up the body, perhaps concentrating on the hips and waist, ask them to imagine they are using an invisible hula hoop and the only way to keep it from falling is long, slow circles. All this can be done in a minimal space...until the arms! This is where the little pokes and prods might emerge when they think you are aren't looking, or even if you are! Again, keep things slow and calm. Choose to move arms and hands upwards rather than sidewards if space is limited. Shrugging shoulders and circling them backwards and forwards. For younger children this is a good opportunity to talk about the different body parts, many won't have heard of forearms or shoulder blades. It's also a winner if you are doing the human body as a topic then you can take it a step further, again depending on age and stage. Here you can use the more medical names – humerus, scapula, sternum, patella. It's a great, interactive way to learn and also incorporate some mindful movement into the bargain.

This doesn't need to be a long session; it can be just a couple of minutes or longer. You'll be able to judge if they've had enough, when you start to see them lose interest or get silly or distracted. As with any of these techniques there is no rush. You are aiming to build a toolkit that hopefully they will be able to access themselves as they develop.

Starting slowly and building up is a good way to let them explore what they like and what works for them. Just like adults, they all won't like the same thing but it's so good to hear them say when they have a few tools up their sleeves,

"I used the breathing when I was scared" or "I coloured in to calm down."

Mindful walking can also be done as part of something else. You probably won't have time to take your class out for a mindful walk as often as you might like but there will be times when your whole class have to get somewhere. This is an opportunity to introduce mindful walking. Again, exaggerate slow, mindful movement, feeling their feet on the floor, paying attention to where they are going and what is around them. Depending on how quickly you have to get there, you might want to incorporate it with the Five Things (senses) exercise that I'll explain about later. With practice, mindful walking can mean they arrive grounded, calm and ready for whatever the next activity is, whether that's assembly, PE, lunch or something else. If you already have to get somewhere anyway, you might as well use the time to add some mindfulness to their day.

Chapter 5

Mandalas and Colouring

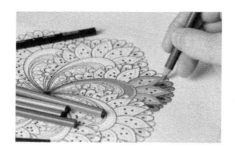

It's hard not to notice, how in recent years there has been an explosion of mindful colouring books which are sold as calming and relaxing activities that reduce stress. And they certainly hit the spot for many adults and children. Often, these books are themed and there is considerable choice and much fun to be had when choosing one. Some of these books are based on more long-established mandala patterns which originate from Hinduism, Buddhism and Jainism traditions. The Sanskrit word for mandala translates to "circle" and they have been used as a spiritual symbol for prayer and meditation. Now, their use tends to be more secular but do tread carefully before introducing these more traditional patterns as some parents or schools may perceive them as religious symbols and object to their use. There are still plenty of useful mindful colouring pages that you can use including many that are free if you search for them online.

To get the most out of using mandalas and colouring and to maximise calm and tranquillity in the classroom make sure you set the scene. As with everything, take into account age and stage of the children you are working with. Make sure they all have a selection of coloured pencils, pens or crayons and try to reduce any movement once the activity has started. It's good to set an intention and many children will be used to the term "learning intention" or "lesson target" which can be as simple as "to feel calm and relaxed." You don't have to mention the word intention but do state what you are hoping they will get from it or, if they are older, they can come up with their own intention. It's good to have a selection of pictures or mandalas but if you are doing it with a whole class giving them a choice can sometimes be tricky if they all want the same one! I usually hand the sheets out face down, randomly and explain what we are going to do. Emphasise the need to stay in their seat and use just what colours they have chosen or share quietly with a partner without talking. You might want to start the exercise with a "Count to Calm" or "Grounding" exercise.

When everyone is ready, ask them to turn the sheet over and just look at it. Noticing the whole pattern, are there patterns or shapes within each other? Do they recognise any? Think about the first colour they are going to choose and where on the pattern will they start? Will it be in the centre or from the outside in? Do they think they will colour lightly or press harder? How does the pattern make them feel? Is it swirly or straight? Remind them to take some mindful breaths in and out. Again, this is very much age and stage related, younger children will need less chat, although you'll be surprised how they settle and focus. Stay calm and gently discourage any excessive talking or whispering. Once they are all colouring it's good to introduce some mindful music – again an online search will yield a vast array of free accessible music. Have it ready to just press play and keep the volume low this will also help to discourage chatter. It's surprising, even with very young children how long they can remain focused when doing this activity.

You will know when the activity is about to expire, either because the young people have reached a natural end to focusing and are becoming restless or because it is the end of a lesson. Keep the atmosphere calm as they mindfully pack away. It's good for them to keep the mandala/colouring in their desk or tray and you can encourage them to come back to it if they are a "fast finisher" or perhaps during some free time. It's also a useful tool for any child who is feeling overwhelmed with a particular situation to be directed to a calm place with some coloured pens, pencils or crayons and take a few minutes out to settle. You might want to have a selection of sheets in a corner of the classroom that they can choose from during free time. Sometimes, as with all new things, some young people will find it hard to focus and may engage in low level disruption. Ignore as much as is possible and just give gentle reminders about how some people want to do this and it's not fair to disturb them. If it becomes a regular feature in your classroom, it's amazing to see how, with time and patience, it becomes a self-regulating tool for many children. If there are neurodivergent young people in your class they may choose to use ear defenders or headphones if the music is not to their taste.

Chapter 6

Mindful Eating and Drinking

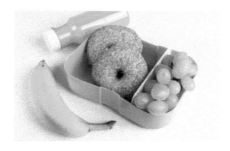

At some point in the school day, young people will need to eat and drink, whether that's a snack, packed lunch or school lunch. This is a great opportunity to teach mindfulness. It can also tie in beautifully with the curriculum in terms of healthy eating, food and technology, farming and many other topics and projects. The aim of the exercise as always is to slow down and be in the present moment. Pre pandemic, this was always a good one to do with a whole class with the same food and my preferred choice was always fruit – usually a strawberry, or sometimes chocolate. Now, it's often better to use the young people's own snack or lunch. Try not to be judgemental there will be a good mixture of just about everything from the healthiest fruit to the unhealthiest combinations of sweet, salty and fatty snacks. Again, as with everything, this is age and stage appropriate in terms of duration and information. This meditation also lends itself to both sensory writing and art. You can do some great follow up lessons adding in more adventurous vocabulary to describe the taste and texture of what they have eaten or drunk. This can also be applied to what they have drawn, painted or sculpted.

As always, set the scene and make sure that hands are washed before handling food. Start by saying how we all rush our food because we're often busy and have to eat something fast so we can get on to the next thing we have to do. Today we are going to do the very opposite and take our time and really appreciate the food we have. A quick glance around the class will give you an idea of what they have in front of them. Don't be daunted that they don't all have the same. You may have to have something available to discreetly offer to those who don't have anything at all. Then, ask them all to put their food in front of them without touching it for now. Take some deep breaths or Count to Calm or ground them before you start.

Now, ask them to just look carefully, without touching whatever their snack or food is. Notice what shape and size it is. Is it in a wrapper, skin, packet or box? This is good for young children to identify shapes and colour; young people and teens might focus more on packaging and the environment. Next let them pick the food up and explore with their hands only! Again, ask them what it feels like: hard, soft, squishy? Turn it over and look at every part of it, is it the same colour all over or different shades? Does it feel rough or smooth, even or bumpy? Is there a stalk or a raisin or chocolate chip poking out? Watch for sneaky pickers! This is a great way to build and extend vocabulary. Next, ask them to listen. This is where the crisp and chocolate fans get the best deal as they rustle their packets! For the next sense, smell, you need to have a quick look round for what your young people have. Ask them to open a small corner if it's a packet or wrapper, not the whole thing. Then encourage them to smell what's inside. The fruit lovers can smell their fruit and see if they can pick out any smell from it. Again, a fantastic way of building and developing vocabulary. You might want to write some of them down on a whiteboard or word wall so they can use them again for writing. Now comes the best bit...almost!

The packets and wrappers can be fully opened. There's often lots of good-natured moans and groans and accusations of torture at this stage. Very small children will probably not have spent so much time in the build-up to eating something. Young people and teens are usually champing at the bit by this time – as with everything, use your judgment as to how long or short this meditation is. You can always redo it and build up stamina! The next stage involves taking the tiniest bite, not a full-blown mouthful. Again, encourage them to notice texture and taste. Is it sweet, sour, salty? Does it melt? Is it crunchy? How does it feel in their mouth? Food can evoke very strong memories; does it remind them of when they last ate it? Who with? You will know your young people and their backgrounds so be careful about triggers. Bear in mind neurodivergent young people who may be triggered by certain senses. It is one of the benefits of them using their own food and also, as always, be aware of allergies and intolerances. Epi-pen aware!

Once they have had a tiny taste you can put them out of their misery by encouraging them to take a bigger bite but still eating slowly and mindfully. Noticing tastes and textures, are there more flavours the more they eat? Encourage and record vocabulary so that you can use it in other lessons. It's good to finish the meditation with gratitude. Ask them to be grateful for; Who provided it, who bought it? Where did it come from? Then consider being grateful to those who grew it, picked it, packed it, shipped it, unpacked it, put it on shelves, wrapped it, sold it...the list is endless. It can also lead to some fantastic discussions about source, carbon footprint, child labour, minimum wage, health, availability. Some fascinating topics that stretch through the curriculum and beyond. I apologise again for using the term 'age and stage' but as you know, there is a vast difference between very small children, young people and teens. Know your audience, use your professional judgement and don't worry if it doesn't go how you planned. As we all know lessons often don't. Let the young people be your teacher, follow their lead. Take it slower or faster next time. Add to it, take something out, focus on one particular sense or outcome. Just remember that mindfulness is about being present in the moment not ticking boxes.

You can do this meditation also with drinks. Water is good but again use what the young people have, whether that's milk or juice. Discuss what it feels like to be thirsty. What do the inside of our mouths feel like? Listen to the liquid in its container. Notice its colour. Does it smell? Take a taste...cold, warm, hot? Is it sweet, creamy or sour? How does it feel when they take a long slow drink? Do the flavours or temperature burst into their mouth or is it a slower experience? Again, use this to build vocabulary. It's good for sensory writing eg it's not just nice it's deliciously, mouth wateringly, scrumptious...you get the picture!

Chapter 7

Mindfulness
and Art

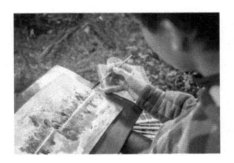

Art is a wonderful way for young people to express themselves. It can also form the basis of some excellent mindful
practices. It can though, be frustrating for some children
and young people who learn at a very early age to doubt
their abilities.

In almost every art lesson, regardless of age, there will
always be at least one adult or young person who says,

"I'm rubbish at art."

Art can be soothing and calming but be aware of those
young people in your classroom who are neurodivergent.
Sometimes colours, textures and the smells of different

media can act as a trigger and provoke a reaction. As with every lesson, knowing the young people in your care goes a long way to avoiding or at least preempting a response that leaves them feeling upset and misunderstood.

As with other lessons and mindfulness sessions, set the scene and set an intention. You can combine a learning intention with a mindfulness intention:

Example - To mindfully explore colour and tone using...whatever medium you choose.

For very young children this can involve something such as discussing actual colours and then introducing terms such as lighter and darker, exploring what happens when one colour is added to another: Does it get lighter or darker? Does it make you feel gloomy or happy? Is it an angry or sad colour? How can we change it into a different shade, colour or hue? Use, the vocabulary you want them to emulate in their descriptions and writing. Discuss, through the senses, what the medium is like; thick, runny, chalky, oily? How does it feel on your fingers? What happens when you spread it out? What happens if you add water? How does it feel and look now? How does it smell? These are things to add in as you continue with the theme of your lesson, whether that's finger painting for the very young, or more complex techniques with young people and teens. You are probably already doing most of these things naturally, so think how much time you will save by using the lesson to impart some mindfulness.

Mindfulness doesn't have to be "another lesson" it should work alongside everything we do so it becomes part and parcel of everyday life.

Chapter 8

Transient Art

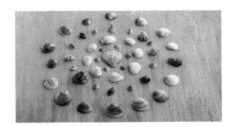

More and more schools are seeing the benefits of being outside in nature. The popularity of Forest Schools has grown exponentially since the concept arrived in the UK in the early 1990's. Many schools now try to incorporate some outdoor learning as often as possible. It is a child/young person-centred approach to learning with massive benefits for health and well-being. There is a plethora of information about it online and a good place to start in the UK is the Forest School Association. (Reference 4)

Being outside in nature is an ideal place to learn about the natural world. It introduces young people to seasons, weather, plants, animals and so much more.

The following session incorporates making outdoor art and can be used with almost anything that can be found outside. If your school is not close to somewhere suitable then you may find yourself scouring beaches, forests and woods at the weekend! All sorts of twigs, leaves, pebbles and shells can be collected and used in the classroom or playground for this lesson. Very young children, and those who are neurodivergent, may have some strong feelings about their art not lasting, so as with everything, prepare them well. Explain that what they are going to make won't be permanent. Perhaps you can take photos of it or they could sketch it so they can remember it. If you prepare them well, hopefully you should be able to avoid a complete meltdown when you have to leave it behind or dismantle it!

The collection process of the natural materials can be a whole mindfulness session in itself. It can begin with mindful walking, being aware of everything around them. Take time to stop and notice everything through their senses. Try to avoid "picking" flowers but any fallen leaves, particularly autumn leaves, are perfect for this activity as are pebbles, twigs and shells. Discuss what they look and feel like. What shape are they? Are they rough or smooth? Long or short, big or small? Throw in some maths as well – is this bigger or smaller than that? As always, age and stage appropriate but make comparisons - is this heavier or lighter? Would it float or sink? Find better adjectives to describe the object. This might be just one lesson with lots of possible follow ups. Once you've exhausted the search, either in terms of time and effort or physically not being able to carry anymore, head to where you want the art to be made.

Another maths activity for younger children is sorting and they can work individually, in pairs or in a small group. Again, you will know them better than anyone and will be the best judge of who and what works together. It's interesting to see how they do sort at this stage and the negotiations and discussion that goes along with it. Encourage chat, listening to how they are grouping things. There is no right or wrong. They can be sorted by colour, shape, size, leaf, stick, rocks, shells or whatever they want. Ask them to use their senses describing everything they notice.

Once sorted you will want to give them the learning and mindful intention. Something like, to make a picture or design using...(whatever they have) mindfully. If they are familiar with mandalas which have been discussed previously, this activity lends itself well to making one. As a form of grounding, ask them to stop and think for a moment before they start. Take some deep breaths, feel the ground under their feet. Think about what they are going to do: Will they start at the centre or the edge? Will it be large or small? Is there a colour scheme? Encourage their use of senses at every stage and speak quietly about patterns and shapes, both natural and those they make. At the end of the session offer a tour around everyone's efforts, reminding them this isn't permanent. Offer to take pictures for a classroom display. Depending on where it is, the art can either be left or dismantled. Pebbles and shells can be reused and you'll be surprised if you have a box in the classroom, how many will go back and make patterns themselves

Chapter 9

Language and Art

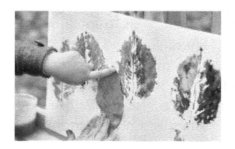

Mindfulness practice lends itself to many different lessons that teachers do in school every day. Using the senses in a mindful way can produce a richness and depth to vocabulary and sentence structure. Even the youngest pupils can learn to "up level" their sentences once they begin to use vocabulary that describes their experiences and emotions through the senses. An increase in technology can be a positive way to record experiences to use later. Often schools will have the use of iPads, tablets or other portable devices that can be used to take photographs or videos for times when it isn't possible to get out and about. These devices can also be invaluable for young people with learning differences who may struggle to either experience some situations first hand or may have difficulty in recording their responses physically. Speech to text has become much better than in the early days. Its use can mean that either very young children, who have not got the writing skills in place, or those with learning differences can record their responses and produce something they are proud of.

One of my former colleagues combined several elements of the curriculum in a fantastic lesson after coming to one of my mindfulness teaching sessions. Just like the transient art lesson previously, the lesson began outside but rather than gathering a lot of resources the young people were encouraged to find one thing that they felt attracted to. So, a leaf or a stone or a twig. They were asked to search mindfully and really think about why they were going to choose their object. Once they had found it they were not to show it to anyone but to keep it safe until they returned to the classroom. The young people were then put into twos and, in turn, asked to describe their object to each other without showing it. The listening partner was encouraged to draw what they thought it was. This can be differentiated according to age and stage. Some were told their object was a leaf or stone, but older children were encouraged to guess from the description. Vocabulary flowed as they found ways to describe their object and questioned shape and size and colour. Then the roles were reversed and the process started again. Encouragement was given for detail, both in drawing and description, and it was stressed that it was the process that was important not the end artistic result. It is fascinating to see how much fine detail they observed that usually would just have passed them by. There were beautiful descriptions of the veins on the leaves, the knots on the branch and even the minibeasts that came along for the ride!

A nice way to combine language and art and foster a love of the natural world at the same time.

Chapter 10

Journaling

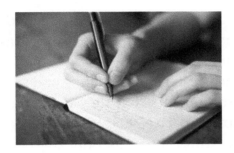

Journaling can be cathartic and a great source of comfort to children and young people of all ages. It can also be the cause of upset, embarrassment and horror if they fall into the wrong hands. This is definitely an activity where you need to know the young people you are working with. There needs to be firm ground rules about who reads them and the importance of privacy, where they are stored and whether they take them home or are simply just done at either home or school. Young people need to feel safe and secure and as educators we need to ensure this is the case.

For young children, journals can be a place to express feelings: drawing, scribbling or just making marks on paper that represent how they feel. For older children and teens, they can be a useful tool not only for expression but for recording and tackling deeper issues. This session may just be about introducing the concept of journaling and possibly providing the materials and then backing off, leaving them to decide if they want to write or not.

If you decide that it is something you want to do as a group or class do make sure you are aware of any triggers that may invoke a response for particular children. Also make sure you are aware of school policies particularly around child protection and safeguarding. This all sounds like gloom and doom and you must be wondering who in their right mind would ever even consider it as an activity! Don't be daunted, just be aware.

A blank canvas can be intimidating and so it is useful to give some starting points that they may want to consider. Don't be tempted to give more than one or two at each session and do stress these are only suggestions. Start by having everything to hand: paper, notebook, coloured pens, pencils. Explain that sometimes it helps us to identify and work through problems or worries or just to see things more easily. As always this should be age and stage appropriate.

With every mindful activity make sure you ground them first in one of the many ways that you now have in your toolkit!

Below are some useful prompts to help you get started. You may have to adjust the wording for some...depending on "age and stage!" Some you may want to avoid with particular young people. It's always good to set a time limit and then it's not a never-ending activity regardless of whether they like it or not. Some young people could spend all day on this while others will have had enough after a few minutes. It can be helpful to play some mindful music very quietly in the background but do be aware and have ear defenders or headphones for those who may not appreciate sound.

Also, don't bombard them with too much. If they start to write an answer to these prompts and get stuck ask them to add 'why' or 'because' to the statement. They may just want to draw or doodle. One of the prompts below is enough at one time, with the possibility of extending it with a why or because. Journals should also never be shared unless the young person chooses to share, and they should never be marked or corrected!

- Today, I feel...because...
- Today, I am grateful for...because...
- Something what makes me happy is...
- Sometimes I worry that...what helps?
- I really enjoy...
- I don't like it when...
- When I (think of any activity) I feel...
- I like the sound, sight, smell, taste, touch of...because...it reminds me of...
- My favourite colour is...because...
- I love it when it snows, rains, when the sun shines...it makes me feel...

These are only suggestions and I'm sure that you will have many more ideas, as will the young people themselves.

Chapter 11

Labyrinths

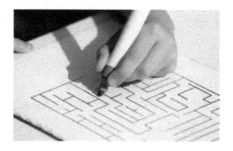

Labyrinths have been around for thousands of years and it is believed that they originated in Ancient Greece. For many they symbolise a journey and there are many ways to "walk" a labyrinth. The labyrinth has been seen to represent a journey and for some it symbolises the journey of life. Sometimes a journey towards peace within oneself, taking into account the highs and lows of life. Some find it mysterious others look on it as a fun type of maze. The difference between a maze and labyrinth being, there is only one way in and out of a labyrinth, no dead ends to get lost in.

Few of us have a life size labyrinth close to us but there are numerous ways to still make the "journey" and get the calming benefits. If you do live close to one though it's well worth a visit to try it out. There are many free paper labyrinths available to download and copy. As with the mandala exercise this can be done individually, with groups or with a whole class. It can be a short calming exercise or a longer deeper exercise, as always depending on age and stage.

Initially set the scene by using one of the grounding exercises and perhaps some quiet mindful music in the background. Check that the young people have everything they need before you begin, to prevent moving about once they are started.

Explain they are going to go on a journey from the entrance of the labyrinth to the centre and back out again. They can do this by just tracing their finger slowly through it or they might want to use a coloured pencil or pen. A highlighter is a good tool for this as generally the tip fills the path space perfectly. This is also a great exercise for fine motor control and younger children like the challenge of making their journey on paper without touching the sides of the labyrinth walls. As with the mandala ask them to use their mindful breathing throughout and remind them that it is a slow journey. When they get to the centre, ask them to think of a special thought, worry or wish that they can leave behind. They can just think it or they can write it on the back of the sheet. When they are ready to leave encourage them to return back through the labyrinth, stopping occasionally to think about their breath or how they are feeling. If you have young people who want to rush it – and it can easily be done in a few seconds – set them a challenge! Encourage them to get in and out of the labyrinth without touching the sides at all using a sharp coloured pencil or pen. Usually those who want to be the fastest are competitive so they are keen to take up the challenge. It's amazing to see a whole class calmly sitting with their labyrinths. Just don't expect it all to happen the first time! As with all the mindful exercises it's important to do them regularly. You'll find that the more you do, the more they'll engage. Expect some silliness and laughs and even a few "this is stupid" comments but if you persevere, they and you, will reap the benefits.

Paper labyrinths are not the only option but they are cheap and easily accessible. Another option is for the young people to make their own. This can be a hand drawn paper version or as with the mandalas and transient art, out of anything they can find. For older students there are many ways of introducing this in a number of subjects and extra-curricular clubs: design technology, art or gardening. The school may even want to invest in making a larger more permanent feature. That could be a project for particular age groups although space might be a drawback. It's worth discussing with them and possibly setting a challenge as to how many versions of a labyrinth they can come up with. Lots of opportunities for extending vocabulary, sharing points of view and debating!

Chapter 12

Gratitude

Gratitude is more than just being thankful for what we have, it's about making a conscious effort to express our appreciation of someone or something. It helps us to shift our focus from ourselves and become more positive about what we have in our lives. For those of you who are interested there are many examples of studies undertaken to show how gratitude has a positive effect on social, emotional, psychological and physical wellbeing. Even Charles Dickens appears to have some understanding of its benefits!

"Reflect on your present blessings, on which every man has many, not on your past misfortunes, of which all men have some."

So, how can we incorporate gratitude into school life? As always, age and stage appropriate, but even the youngest of our children can be taught not just to say thank you, but to be truly grateful for everyday small events or things. As mentioned in the mindful eating and drinking section, just spending a few minutes thinking about where their snack came from or who made it can have a positive impact.

Rather than a nod to good manners and a quick thank you, (never to be discouraged!) just take it a small step further.

Things to ask - What are we grateful for today? Our warm coat, sunscreen, running outside, a water bottle for drinking from? There are lots of everyday situations and occurrences that we take for granted and it is only when we consciously reflect on them that we fully appreciate the time, effort, and the impact they have made on us. Children can be encouraged to draw or write a note of thanks to someone or even just say thank you but with a real understanding of the difference the action or object has made to them.

A sixth form college in Calderdale, Halifax (UK) has adopted a two-minute silence every morning for reflection. This involves all the students and staff. They are told it is two minutes in a busy day when they can give thanks, pray or just be still. If this isn't something your whole school or college feel they want to adopt it can be done with a registration group, a whole class practice, or a subject specific class that you teach. It could also be a way to end a day, reflecting on something positive that has been experienced. These are only suggestions I'm sure you will come up with many more, as will the young people you teach.

Chapter 13

5 4 3 2 1

This is a nice exercise to do both indoors and outside and it's also an interesting one to repeat often, since everything changes depending on location, time, season, weather and mood!

This is good for all age groups and you can adapt the timing accordingly. First, as always, make sure the young people are grounded and explain they will be standing or sitting still for this exercise, not wandering about. Then, ask them to look around carefully and mindfully and choose 5 things they can see. Timing with this will very definitely be around age and stage. This isn't just about quickly finding five things, encourage them to notice one at a time. Ask them to think of its size, shape and colour. Repeat this until they have seen five things in their environment. Then ask them to close their eyes if they can for the rest of the exercise, but do bear in mind that some may not like this. If this is the case explain how important it is not to make eye contact or put someone else off. Then ask them to listen for four different sounds, again not rushing but taking time to identify what the sound is, where it is coming from, is it loud or soft, near or far. Next ask them to smell three different things if they can, this will be easy or more difficult depending on when or where it's done. Then, ask them to find two things they can touch, again reminding them they can't move about but they can touch the ground, their hair, clothes or skin, thinking about what each one in turn feels like. Finally, ask them to taste one thing – this might be trickier but suggestions can include their last snack or drink or you might want to encourage them to take a sip from their water bottle and notice what they're drinking, is it cold or warm, sweet or just water?

The order of the senses doesn't matter, if you are outside for example, you may want them to move mindfully for part of this exercise. Remind them this means moving slowly and really noticing what that feels like. Ask them to find different textures to touch or see, so you can easily make touch the first option of the five. Once completed that can just be the end of the exercise or you can encourage discussion, comparisons, extending vocabulary and recording what they have done in some way. That may take the form of a journal exercise, a drawing or a piece of sensory creative writing. If they, and you, are using their senses then it could be wise to capitalise on it and make use of it in a lesson if you can.

Chapter 14

Four Point or Square Breathing

This is another meditation for the tool box that can easily be adapted and used for all kinds of situations. It works well with the very youngest primary school children, right through to college and university students and adults too.

As ever, age and stage appropriate is always the mantra as is grounding yourself and the young people before you begin.

Help younger children identify something in the room that has four sides. It doesn't need to be a square. A window, door, whiteboard, book, paper are all usually available. They just need to be able to see something while you demonstrate. Remember some find visualisation difficult so it is good to give them examples.

Next, tell them you are going to start in the bottom left-hand corner of the shape and take a deep breath in as their eyes travel up to the top left-hand corner as you count one. When you arrive at the top corner, take a pause, but there should be no breath holding. Then slowly, release the breath, eyes travelling across the object to the top right-hand corner, counting two. Again, take a pause before taking the next deep breath eyes moving down to the bottom right-hand corner counting three. Pause again, before releasing the breath slowly as eyes follow back to the beginning as you count four. This can be repeated as many times as needed. Remember to emphasise the slowness and the breathing as it's being done. Once they know what they are doing they can close their eyes and visualise the four points. This is really useful for those times when feeling overwhelmed can result in anxiety, fear and loss of performance especially in exams. It can take 30 seconds or longer depending on time constraints and no one need know they are doing it (Reference 5).

Chapter 15

Rainbow Breathing

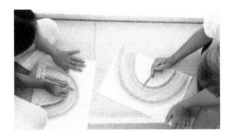

This is a lovely practice to do with younger children and you can extend it by getting them to draw and colour a rainbow before they begin so that they can use it as a prop. If you don't have time before the session, they can draw it afterwards and use it the next time. You might even want to have a whole class activity and make a beautiful rainbow display.

Begin with a short grounding exercise and then either show them a rainbow picture or get them to use the ones they've made.

Start by demonstrating a deep breath and following the arc of the rainbow by tracing a finger or their eyes along the red arc. As they reach the top they can pause briefly, no breath holding, before letting out a long slow breath down to the bottom of the rainbow.

Do the same with each rainbow colour in order. This is a great way of teaching or reinforcing colours to very young children too.

One round might be enough but you can repeat it as many times as it takes to restore calm! (Reference 6)

Chapter 16

Feeling the Breath, Starfish Breathing

Again, this is a lovely practice to use with very young children. It's a nice introduction to feeling the breath and what happens in their body when they do. We don't often think about our breath and where we feel it so this can be a good practical demonstration that children can relate to. As ever begin by grounding them with an activity from your toolkit. Explain that we all sometimes feel grumpy, upset, angry, tired etc and that all these emotions are normal. Then practice some slow breathing in and out. You can explain that breathing in can be like smelling a beautiful flower or their very favourite smell, maybe chocolate, pizza or something else they can imagine. The main thing is that it is slow and mindful. When they breathe out it's like blowing one single candle out on a birthday cake – not a big blow but a long soft gentle one. Before they take the next breath ask them to put their hands on their tummy and when they breathe notice what happens to their hands. They should notice that they go up and down. Encourage them to try this at home in bed if they can't sleep, maybe resting their special toy on their tummy and noticing how it moves with each breath.

Starfish breathing is an easy way for very young children to understand the movement of their breath. Begin by asking them to spread their fingers out in front of them just like a starfish. Then, ask them to take a breath in and use their index finger from the other hand to trace from the base of the thumb, just at the wrist, to the top of the thumb. Brief pause at the top, but no breath holding, and then moving their finger down the other side of the thumb to the space between the thumb and index finger. Another pause, before a breath in and they travel up to the top of the next finger and so on. This can be repeated as many times as needed and once it's been taught children can be directed to use it independently when they need to feel calm. Again, a pre or post activity might involve drawing and mindfully colouring their starfish! (Reference 7)

Chapter 17

Making a Glitter Jar

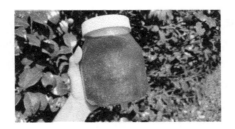

This is a well-loved activity and I'm always pleasantly surprised that older children and young people enjoy it as much as the younger ones. It's a visual way of helping them to be aware of, and how to regulate, feelings and emotions. It's good to have "one you made earlier" for this, as it not only helps them to see the end result, but you can also do a demonstration of mindfulness before you start the activity.

Begin by talking about how sometimes our minds are so full of thoughts and ideas, things we have to do or not do, places we have to be, things we have to get or achieve, that we can feel overwhelmed and stressed. Often, we're trying to do too many things at once. As you are speaking, turn the jar upside down and side to side to show the movement of glitter in the jar. Notice how it whirls and swirls like a maelstrom. Explain this is what our head can feel like when full of thoughts and emotions and what we need is to find a way to help this. It's important to say here that mindfulness isn't about emptying our mind or controlling our thoughts, it's about not letting our thoughts and actions control us. Talk about sitting quietly and focusing on our breathing, perhaps using one of the techniques we have used before, then our thoughts begin to settle and we become calmer. Show the glitter beginning to slow and settle too in the jar but explain there will always be one or two "thoughts" gently floating and that's ok.

Then the young people can make their own glitter jar. Please be aware of the safety aspects of young children and glass for this activity. It's a good idea for parents or carers to collect the jar along with their child at the end of the school day. Suggest that older children and young people wrap it in a towel or some other suitable padding and make sure the lid is screwed on tight. It can be good to have a "class" glitter jar that can be kept on a shelf safely and used by you with the whole class for mindful activities or by an individual child in a quiet space when they need to feel calm and safe.

You will need: -

- Glass jar with a firm lid
- Water
- Selection of food colourings
- Glitter and/or coloured sequins – it is possible to get biodegradable but is more expensive
- Glycerine or pva glue
- Pipettes (optional but they do make life easier!)

Begin by filling the jars with water, almost to the brim. Depending on age and stage this can mean them filling the jars themselves at the sink under supervision or may mean you and an assistant taking a jug of water and filling them for them. As always you know the young people you are working with best.

The next stage is choosing the colour; try to have a few different food colourings to demonstrate. It's also a good lesson to talk about shades of colour, discussing how a little makes lighter colours, more makes darker colours. If you're feeling brave, mix colours!

Pipettes are great for adding one or two drops at a time. I always make the rule that they have to stick with the water they have so if they add too much it can't be changed. This saves an endless trek to the sink and a queue of children wanting to change colours every few minutes. You might be more tolerant though!

Tell them to start with just a drop and add slowly until they are happy with the colour. Food colouring does stain so please make sure you have taken reasonable precautions and avoid it coming into contact with clothes and skin. It does eventually wash off skin but clothes not so much and you don't want a line of unhappy parents demanding the school pay for new clothes!

When they are happy with the colour then they can add glitter. Again, if you're lucky enough to have a choice of colours ask them to think carefully because it cannot be undone or started again. A couple of teaspoons of glitter is usually enough although you and they can experiment with more or less depending on your budget and availability. If you have any sequins they can also be added at this stage. Finally, add a couple of drops of either glycerine or pva glue into the jar. You will know your young people and can decide whether they can do this themselves or if you or an assistant does it for them. The purpose of this is to stop the glitter from clumping and just plummeting to the bottom of the jar when it's shaken up. Finally, screw the tops on the jars tightly. Once everything is cleared away it's good to have them all sit with their jars and shake them, reminding them to think of their breath and slowing down as they watch the glitter settle. You might like to play some calming mindful music as they, and you, enjoy a few mindful minutes. The jars can be decorated using permanent markers if you wish. This can be another activity in itself but do be careful they don't add so much decoration that they can't see the glitter as this will defeat the purpose. The jars are just as good without decoration and they may be happy to leave them as they are.

Chapter 18

Making a Stress Toy

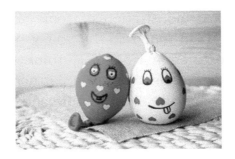

There has been an explosion in so-called fidget toys and stress relieving objects, many of which can be seen as more of a hindrance than a help in the classroom. Sometimes it feels like everyone needs one and those of us who were around when the finger spinners and decompression toys were at their height could be forgiven for completely ignoring this section altogether! For some children and young people though, stress toys can be a lifeline and a much-needed strategy for focusing attention by keeping hands busy during a potential flashpoint, or just as a comfort.

These can be made with individuals, small groups and whole classes as well as after school and extracurricular clubs.

You will need: -

- Selection of coloured deflated balloons (regular round shape)
- Dried rice, lentils, quinoa, flour, fine sand or other dried ingredients
- Funnels
- Permanent markers

Begin with a demonstration of some you have made earlier, passing them round so the young people can feel the different textures. Ask them to think how each one feels, perhaps describing them to a partner. This is good for exploring vocabulary about texture and size as well as guessing what might be in each one. Once they have all had the opportunity to feel the balloons ask them to think about which texture, they would like to choose for their own. A word to the wise– the flour filled balloons can prove quite messy if they burst, so maybe exercise some ground rules and caution. Obviously, as always, you know your class best and can judge whether you offer flour or not! Once they have chosen their balloon and filling you might want to group them on tables so that each table has just one of the fillings. This saves on a lot of passing about and spillages.

Demonstrate how to attach the funnel to the base of the balloon and then slowly and gently add whichever dried ingredient they have chosen. Suggest they cooperate and assist each other with fixing the funnel on the balloon. Encourage them to stop and feel how firm or soft the balloon is and how much more they want to add. Ask them to think about what will happen the more they add. Will it be harder, softer or stronger. Remind them that they have to tie a knot in the balloon when they have filled it enough. Depending on age and stage they may need help with this and an extra pair of hands from a classroom assistant or volunteer could be welcome.

Once their balloon is tied securely, give them chance to explore it themselves. Perhaps comparing theirs with a partner's, again extending vocabulary to describe exactly what they feel. Next, they can use the permanent marker pens to decorate the balloon. There isn't a lot of room on a deflated balloon so this won't take them long. Some might like to add a couple of words such as "breathe," "calm" or "relax;" others might draw something symbolic to them, like a flower or other pattern. If they have used the 5 4 3 2 1 breathing technique from earlier, adding these numbers can serve as a reminder of something to do while using their stress toy.

The stress toys are small enough to carry around in a pocket and used discreetly when needed. They can be used in class or taken home. It's good to have one or two available in the classroom that can be used by anyone if they've left theirs at home.

Chapter 19

Bubbles and Windmills

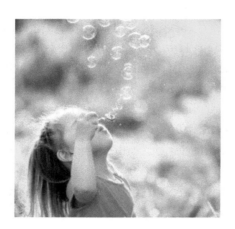

This is a great activity to do with very young children as it provides a visual representation of the power of their breath. Breathing is the basis of mindfulness and getting even very young children to focus on their breath shouldn't be underestimated. Bubbles and windmills are fun, cheap ways of experimenting with breath. Use them to demonstrate long, slow breaths, noticing what happens when we purse our lips in different ways. Get them to try blowing bigger bubbles, discussing long, short, controlled breathing. Demonstrate more powerful breathing with the windmills. Knowing the children you are working with will help you decide if they work best individually, in pairs or small groups or whether you need to keep it as something you do all together. Again, don't underestimate the language activities that this can produce. Talk about bigger, smaller, spherical, transparent, translucent. Practise breathing in and out together. Notice size and shapes with the bubbles or fast and slow with the windmills. Pretend the windmill is a beautiful flower and breathe in as if you're smelling its scent, breathing out enough to blow one birthday candle out on a cake. Vary the length and strength of the breath. Experiment, have fun and they will too. Some schools have a buddy system where younger children are partnered up with older year groups, this is a lovely activity for them to share together. It also enables older children to engage with their breath in a cool way. Even teens have been known to enjoy a bubble session so don't write it off as a childish activity if you teach older students. We all need to get in touch with our inner child sometimes!

Chapter 20

Final Reflections

We live in a busy world where success is often defined by how much we can do in as little time as possible. This isn't sustainable and isn't good for our mental health and certainly not good for our young people's mental health. The pandemic showed us all how fragile we can be. The knock-on effects of those months in lockdown continue to live with us, and I suspect will for a good number of years. One of the greatest gifts we can give to future generations is a toolbox that they can use again and again when they feel anxious, worried and generally overwhelmed by what life is throwing at them. If we can sow the seeds of self-care when they are young then hopefully, they will take these skills and tools with them throughout their lives. They have to know that there is more to life than constantly feeling overwhelmed with "doing". We are human beings and need to learn how to just be. That's not to say striving to achieve is bad but it needs to be balanced so that our young people can learn resilience and self-respect. They need to recognise what's going on within and what tools and strategies they can use to help them achieve their best selves.

There are many more mindful techniques, exercises and strategies that we can teach our young people; the ones in this book are just a selection of what's out there. They aren't new and I certainly don't claim to have invented any of them. Most of them can be found through a good web search but hopefully I have managed to pull enough together to save you some time. The ideas in this book are not intended to replace courses or programmes that are already in place in your schools, but I hope that they can complement what's there and be fitted easily into a school day. I can honestly say I have used all of them, all successfully, although not necessarily first time!

It takes time to build up a mindfulness practice and I would urge any of you who teach, or are expected to teach mindfulness, to make sure you do practice what you preach. It's no use playing a mindfulness meditation and then sitting at the back of the room marking a pile of books, tempting as that is. The young people will see you aren't invested in it and therefore why should they be?

Apart from anything else you really don't want to miss out on the benefits that can be gained from practising mindfulness. Good Luck, I hope this goes a small way to making your life a little easier.

References

1 Mindfulness for Kids - https://www.mindful.org/mindfulness-for-kids/

2 Chris Maxwell - https://insighttimer.com/mindfuliveschris

3 Count To Calm - https://insighttimer.com/mindfuliveschris/guided-meditations/count-to-calm

4 What is Forest School? - https://forestschoolassociation.org/what-is-forest-school/

5 Square Breathing for Challenging Times - https://insight-timer.com/mindfuliveschris/guided-meditations/square-breathing-for-challenging-times

6 Rainbow Breathing for Children - https://insighttimer.com/mindfuliveschris/guided-meditations/rainbow-meditation-for-children

7 Starfish Breathing for Kids - https://insighttimer.com/mindfuliveschris/guided-meditations/star-fish-breathing-for-kids

Acknowledgements

This book would not have been possible without the time, patience and editing skills of both Irene Williams and Angela Sturgeon. I can't thank you enough for the hours spent helping me with this.

To Craig Sturgeon, without your IT skills I would have fallen at the first fence!

To my daughter Suzy for her honest opinions, insight and grounding comments, especially in the editing process!

To my teaching colleagues around the world who are still out there in various schools and colleges, doing their best to bring mindfulness to the next generations.

And finally, to the many hundreds, if not thousands, of children that I have had the privilege to work with over the years, you have been my greatest teachers. I hope I have been able to pass on something useful that you can use for the rest of your lives.

Milton Keynes UK
Ingram Content Group UK Ltd.
UKHW021911091023
430253UK00005B/7